Contents:

Introduction

I decided to write this book because I have been looking after my mother for the last seven years with the help of Social Services – it is a subject that is close to my heart. During this time I have gained valuable knowledge at a personal level about what is involved in caring for an elderly person with dementia. It is my sincere hope that this book will be useful to people in the same situation as mine, and maybe solve some problems they might face.

Looking after an elderly relative is a personal decision that a lot of people might have to face in the future. People are living longer than before. A century ago the average life span was 40 - 45. Now it is forecast to be over 85 by the year 2020. The government has a problem about how to pay for social care if a large percentage need help to stay independent at home - or a more expensive problem if they are going to fund care in care homes.

THE AVERAGE COST FOR A RESIDENT IN A CARE HOME IS £400 A PER WEEK. In some care homes this figure could be as much as £1,000. That is an average of £30,000 annually just to look after an elderly person in a care home.

The government want to give people the option of living at home which is the cheaper and better option. And the help is out there, but I feel this only works if a relative or a neighbour can give some of their time to help out voluntarily. This is something I have done. You can call it sacrifice as well. A sacrifice where you have to resign from that secure job you had; a sacrifice where you have to cut back on your social time. This means your finances are going to be seriously dented. Serious consideration needs to be made before taking up your role as a carer.

If the decision is made to become a carer for your relative, there is help out there. Hopefully, this book will help you understand the assistance you can receive and the things you can do yourself to solve problems.

In this book all the relevant chapters are titled so you can jump to the subject matter that interests you. It is not intended that you should necessarily read this book from first page to last.

How to Get Help

In the beginning I was only giving minor help to my mother; help such as giving her a lift to the doctor or the local health clinic. Generally this is how it starts for most carers. You begin by giving minor help, then gradually the help becomes more frequent and before long you find yourself devoting more and more time to caring for them.

It came to the point where I had to cancel my available overtime at my work place and cut back on some of my social time because it was not safe to leave my mother alone for long periods. The first signs of problems were when she began to forget to take the key when going out. Anybody can forget to take the key once in a while, but this was happening on a regular basis. To combat this problem, I made her a "Key Necklace." The front door key was attached to a long piece of string to make the necklace.

The second problem was her forgetting to switch off the cooker. Twice my mother went out to talk to a neighbour and they noticed smoke coming out of the window and they rushed in to switch off the cooker. To solve this problem I would leave microwavable food for her to heat up for lunch. Later I managed to secure the Meals on Wheels service - they deliver ready to eat, hot meals to your doorstep. I discuss the Meals on Wheels service in more detail later in this book.

If you find problems happening and you need help to cope, the first thing to do is contact your doctor who can register your parent with the Social Services. They will make an assessment of what help is needed. You can also contact them directly, but the official way is through your local GP.

Social Services

The Social Services are a department set up to look after members of society who are vulnerable; including the young, the old, disabled people and those who for health reasons, cannot help themselves, and who might need specialist care. The service was originally set up in 1948 as part of the welfare system which was founded to provided health and social care for all, regardless if they were rich or poor. Before that there was the Poor Law of 1834 which provided only for the very needy and created systemically harsh conditions so only the desperate would apply. The Dickensian work houses were meant for the disadvantaged young and old and these poor wretches were once famously depicted in a poster as receiving worse treatment than slaves.

I have only given you this brief history so there is a understanding of how things were in the past; I'll be briefly covering the present system and how social care might change in the future in England. (In Scotland the laws are separate). At present the Social Services are free at the point of delivery, but in England, if you have capital over £23,250, you have to pay for the services until your capital reduces to below £23,250.

Below are the criteria set out for savings:

(2010 April) England - £23,250

(2010 April) Wales - £22,000

Scotland - Free regardless of your savings

(Savings below £14,250 are ignored. If someone has savings that are in between these figures, they are expected to contribute towards their care costs.)

What help is provided is dependent on the carer's circumstances. If there is a problem you cannot cope with and need advice or help, you can contact the Social Services directly. Each council has its own Social Services department. The official way to seek help is to contact your doctor and ask him/her to refer you to the Social Services. If you have been in hospital, you can ask for help from the Social Services if you cannot cope when you are discharged. However, they don't always tell you there is extra help for you to recover at home - even if it is apparent that you need it.

What happened when my mother required medical care illustrates the fact that obtaining help is not always that easy. In my mother's case she was in terrible pain due to an ulcer on her leg. She was not able to walk to the bathroom. I had to provide a bucket for her. The pain got so bad that even standing became unbearable. My mother couldn't sleep with the acute pain. This meant that I spent maybe 24-36 hours with only couple of hours sleep whilst looking after her. Eventually at 5am, I decided to call her an ambulance. When the ambulance crew refused to take her to the hospital I was shocked. They said it was just a pain in her leg. They also said that the antibiotics she was taking would kick in soon and she would feel better. When I mentioned that she was hardly able to stand or to go to the bathroom, I was told it was a Social Service problem. No explanation was given to me how to receive help from the Social Service and more importantly, how to receive help immediately.

At 9am, as usual, the district nurses came and changed the dressing on her leg. The tendons on her leg were showing through the flesh and my mother was screaming with pain.

The ambulance was called again at 10am. At the insistence of the district nurses, the ambulance crew agreed to take her to the hospital. At the hospital - after three hours of waiting – the doctors said her condition was not critical so they could not admit her.

By this time I was at the point of collapse; with her high blood pressure, her pain and lack of sleep, I am sure my mother was also close to collapsing. I simply said I could not cope; that I needed extra help. On hearing this, the staff quickly called the social worker.

The social worker could see that I was very fatigued and my mother was in a lot of pain. The medical staff did some quick tests to check my mother's mobility and decided to admit her.

It took three months before my mother was well enough to go home. On her return, the Social Services arranged the help and set up the equipment that she required to cope with her condition.

If I hadn't said that I couldn't cope and we were sent home from the hospital, I don't believe either of us would be alive today.

I told you this story to highlight that sometimes things can become critical before you can receive help. It is important to insist that you need help when you approach your GP or contact the Social Services directly. Basically, you need to make as much fuss as you can for them to take you seriously.

<u>Health Practitioners</u> (and Social Care Workers in the Community)

Below is a list of the health practitioners and Social Service departments in the community. All of them are interconnected and communicate with each other to decide what help to give or even reduce their help if not needed any more. Ideally, the referral should be from your GP or you can contact the Social Service directly. The list is in order of importance.

General Practitioners

Your local doctor can refer you to the Social Services if you are vulnerable and need extra help. He/she can also refer you to the district nurses in your community if you need nursing care. Care such as giving insulin injections or applying dressings for wounds. If necessary they can refer you to a specialist if they cannot solve your medical problem.

Mental Health Department

As the name indicates, they specialise in matters of the mind. They care for people who suffer from dementia, schizophrenia and other mental illnesses. They can recommend what treatment is best. They are in direct contact with the Social Services and will advise them about what help a patient might need. Referral is from your GP.

Social Workers

Social workers assess people who are vulnerable and decide what care plan is needed for them. They work under the auspices of the local council. They deal with those who are very young, the mentally ill and the elderly. In hospitals there should be social workers available at all times. If you are going to be discharged and there are concerns about how you are going to cope at home, you should ask to speak to a social worker.

District Nurses

They work in the community visiting people who need nursing care which can be safely administered at home.

Occupational Therapists

Occupational therapists are health professionals who help patients to regain their pre-illness/injury abilities. They might typically help people to dress themselves, achieve mobility in the home and generally perform every-day tasks. They can recommend equipment for a patient to help with their mobility, and give them exercises to improve their mobility. They work in liaison with the social worker and can recommend if a patient needs extra help from a professional carer. In hospital there should be an occupational therapist who will assess a patient's mobility. If there are concerns they will try to improve the situation through giving the patient relevant exercise routines. They can also prescribe specialist equipment or extra help at home when a patient is discharged from hospital.

Care Agencies

They employ trained carers to visit homes to give specialised help for the vulnerable and disabled. They get their clients through the Social Services department. Some people who can afford it, have a private contract with the agency to hire carers who will visit their home to help them with the essential things they can no longer do themselves. A good care agency will regularly send their carers on training courses. They will also ensure that potential employees are checked by the Criminal Records Bureau to make sure they don't have a criminal record.

Carers

A professional carer is someone trained to take care of people who have lost their independence and need extra help. They regularly attend courses dealing with different aspects of care and need a certificate in Social Care to gain employment. They will also undergo Criminal Records Bureau checks.

Here is a flow chart showing how GPs, Health Practitioners and the Social Services communicate with each other to effectively administer help.

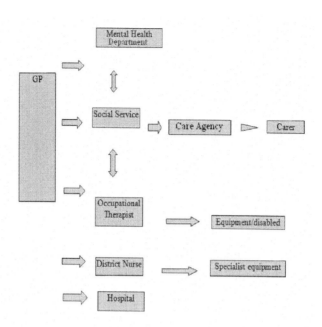

Benefits

Carer's Allowance

If you are 16 years of age or older and you are looking after someone who needs care – typically, a relative - for more than 35 hours a week, you are entitled to Carer's Allowance of £55.55 per week (October 2011). For you to be eligible for Carer's Allowance, the person you are looking after has to be receiving one of the following benefits:

- Disability Allowance

- Attendance Allowance

- Constant Attendance Allowance

You cannot get Carers Allowance if you are in full-time education or earning more than £100 a week after tax.

Income Support

Full-time carers should be eligible for income support, but it depends on their savings and their age on how much they get. There are more ancillary benefits connected to income support than just the Carer's Allowance. Some of these benefits are listed below:

Free dental care

Free prescriptions

Free eye test every two years

Concessions on selected mini module courses in college

Concessions on bus fare

Disability Living Allowance: A benefit for people who have mobility impairment which includes mental illness and learning difficulty.

Attendance Allowance: A benefit for people over the age of 65 who have care needs because of a physical disability, mental illness or age related frailty.

Benefits Office Contact Numbers

Telephone: 0800 055 6688
Text phone: 0800 023 4888
You can also make your claim in Welsh. Telephone: 0800 012 1888

Home Help – Who Pays?

Where day-to-day tasks such as shopping, bathing, collecting your pension etc. become a problem, the Social Services provide you with a home help so you can live independently at home.

There are certain problems that family members or trusted neighbours might be able to solve. However, in situations where they cannot always be relied on to be available 24/7, the Social Services can assess what your needs are and decide if you are eligible to receive help. Below are the three main forms of assistance they can give.

Bathing - If you have suffered a stroke or are incapacitated because of injury or a serious illness and cannot bath yourself, Social Services can provide a trained carer to help bath you at home

Shopping - Social Services can provide a carer to do your shopping

Money - A carer can collect your pension and/or other benefits

Who Pays for Home Care?

If you have savings above the criteria set out by the government, you have to pay for your care.

Savings levels:

(2010 April) England - £23,250

(2010 April) Wales - £22,000

Scotland - Free regardless of your savings

If your savings are below £14,250 or subsequently fall below this figure, the local authority will pay for your care. If your savings are between £14,250 and the levels set out above, you are expected to make a contribution towards your care costs.

Note: If you are ineligible for home care because you don't meet the governments' criteria on savings, certain problems can be solved if you have use of the Internet. Below are the two main online resources available to people who are unable to venture out easily.

Internet shopping with home delivery is now widely available. The major UK supermarket chains offer cheap – to your doorstep - delivery services, provided you spend an average of £20 (or more) on each order.

Banking transactions can be undertaken online (or via telephone banking), making it simple to pay your bills without having to leave home.

Home Adaptions for the Disabled

There is a disability grant available to modify the home to suit the disabled person. The basic modifications are to put holding bars in place in the corridors or where there are steps to negotiate.

Here are five examples of modifications covered by the grant:

1) Depending on the level of disability, steps can be modified into ramps for wheel chair use.

2) There are stair lifts for when people are unable to walk up a flight of stairs. They sit on a motorised chair fitted to the bottom of the staircase. With a push of a button the chair will take them to the top of the staircase. Then there is a motorised lift for single steps. This equipment can only be installed if there is space available.

3) The bathroom can be modified into a walk-in shower. Basically there are no steps and it is possible just to wheel the person in using a wheeled shower chair. **Note:** We had this fitted for my mother and it has been very a useful bathing aid. Over the years her walking ability has become worse and without this modification she would only be able to have a strip wash.*

4) Doorways can be widened to cater for ease of access for wheelchairs. Standard doorways are very narrow for wheelchairs. When you have a narrow corridor leading into a room, the space to turn the wheelchair can be very tight. This can be solved by widening the doorway.

5) Lifting hoists can be attached to ceilings. A bar is placed across the ceiling and a motorised pulley system is used to lift the patient from bed to chair or vice versa.

*Strip wash: A flannel is used to wipe the body with soap and water from a bowl.

Meals on Wheels

Meals on Wheels is a service provided by the local council's Social Services department. They deliver frozen meals which can be kept in the freezer to be heated when required. They also deliver hot meals on a daily basis. The Social Services department first has to assess the individual to find out if they are eligible for the service. Meals on Wheels are intended for people who find it difficult to cook for themselves. There might be a charge for the service; how much depends on which local authority is providing the service.

When I was out all day at work, this was a useful service for my mother. She was not able to make a proper meal for herself; she was always cutting her fingers when slicing vegetables and couple of times she forgot to switch off the cooker. Once, a neighbour, an old man, now sadly passed away, saw smoke coming through the window and noticed that my mother was outside. It transpired that she had locked the door forgetting to take the door key. He did a very brave act by climbing through the open window and switching off the cooker.

The Meals on Wheels service meant she no longer had to worry about cooking for herself. She always knew there would be a hot meal delivered for her lunch. I would rate it as a very good service, particularly the choice of meals, punctuality and cost.

Modifying Clothing

In the beginning, when my mother first started to lose her mobility, helping her to change her clothes was straight forward, but when her mobility started to deteriorate it became harder to help her get changed.

What we did was modify her dresses so they were easy to take off and put new ones on. Usually my mother wears kaftans. It is a garment very popular in South East Asia. The cut is similar to a lady's full-length night gown, but the feel and look of the garment is different.

Kaftans are very comfortable loose fitting dresses. Many women choose to wear them for everyday use - both around the house and when they are out and about. They are very practical garments and can even double as night dresses.

To make the dresses easier put on and take off, I asked a local tailor to make cuts at the back from top to bottom and sew on push buttons. The kaftans then became very similar to those garments worn in hospitals by patients who need to undergo surgery.

Here's a drawing of the garment modification.

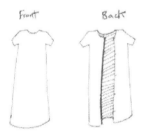

<u>Support Plan</u>

For a full-time carer it is important to have an emergency support plan if suddenly they become ill or for some unforeseen reason they cannot look after their elderly charge.

A list should be drawn-up of people who could act as temporary helpers. A list should also be made of the medications taken, what time to administer medication and past/present medical problems. A third list should be made of daily activities the carer should undertake for the person. If this is not done, particularly for an elderly person suffering from dementia, they may not be able to say what needs to be done for them. This could cause unnecessary suffering or even put their life in danger.

On the following pages you will find examples of the lists mentioned in the last paragraph. If you create similar lists, make sure that every person acting as a temporary carer has access to copies.

Medications for Mr/Mrs..........   **Date:**

	Repeat Medication	Creams
Morning		
Afternoon		
Evening		
Night		

Medical Conditions of Mrs/Mr ....

Daily Routine – 24 Hour Plan for Mr/Mrs..........   Date:

6am-8am	
8am-10am	Brush teeth - Breakfast -
10pm-12pm	
12pm-2pm	
2pm-4pm	
4pm-6pm	
6pm-8pm	
8pm-10pm	
10pm-12am	
12am-2am	
2am-4am	

Emergency Contact Numbers for Mr/Mrs.............

	Name-Telephone	Address-e-mail
Full-time carer		
Next of kin 1		
Next of kin 2		
Care Agency		
Carer (from agency)		
Emergency respite		
Neighbour/volunteer help		
Emergency plumber		
Emergency builder(minor repairs)		
Social service support worker		
GP		
District nurse		
Podiatrist		
Hospital-Consultant		

Ventilation

If you ever find yourself suddenly wheezing for no apparent reason, just opening the window can solve the problem. The oxygen level in the room might have gone down very low. By opening the window you let in more oxygen – this will immediately help you to breathe easier.

Good ventilation in a room is important for health, especially when someone is ill or not feeling very well. Opening a window a couple of times a day, even in the winter time, will let in fresh air. This will make a difference to a person's health and wellbeing. Fresh air carries more oxygen and is electrically charged with positive ions. If a room is poorly ventilated, the oxygen level in the room becomes low which can be particularly dangerous for people who suffer from breathing difficulties caused by conditions such as asthma or pneumonia.

Lighting scented candles in the room of an elderly person or asthma sufferer should be avoided. The candles flame needs oxygen to burn, so you are depleting the oxygen levels in the room. A scented candle can burn for a many hours, so the oxygen levels in the room can steadily become low.

The Humidity of a Room

In winter, keeping the heating on most of the time can make the air in the room very dry. This can dry out skin, and elderly people are very susceptible to dry skin conditions. One way of combating this is to leave a bowl of water in the centre of the room. The evaporating vapour will humidify the room to a certain degree. The second method is to leave washed clothes to dry on radiators. The third method is to switch on a shower for five minutes on a hot setting; then close all windows and turn off any extractor fans. Leave the door of the shower room/bathroom open to allow the steam to circulate throughout the house. The forth method is to leave a window open a few times a day to let in fresh (moist) air.

Respite Care for Carers - Who Pays?

In England and Wales up to eight weeks of respite care for carers is normally available. The respite care is to provide a complete break for the carer. The carer must be a relative or friend, not someone who has a contract (professionally employed) to look after the elderly person's care needs.

Respite care provides temporary residential/nursing care for elderly people who have savings below the criteria allowed by the government. This is when the local authority will pay for the elderly person to be cared for in a care home if they have savings below the following levels:

(2010 April) England- £23,250

(2010 April) Wales - £22,000

Scotland - Free regardless of your savings

(Savings below £14,250 are ignored. If someone has savings that are in between these figures, they are expected to contribute towards their care costs.)

After eight weeks the estate of the elderly person will be taken into account to pay for the care. **But this is only if the care is deemed to be residential, not nursing care.**

Nursing home care - If the care of the elderly person is currently undertaken in hospital and they can be transferred to a nursing home for the management of their illness, the local health authority has a duty to pay for the nursing care.

Residential home care - If the care is deemed residential, meaning care can be met at home with extra help from the local authority and the community nurse, which means the elderly person could be placed in a care home instead of at living at home. Then the person's estate will be taken into account.

Note 1: The local authority normally encourage the carer to take four weeks of respite care instead of the whole eight weeks. This is to save some weeks for emergency situations. When I had a hernia operation, I had to put my mother in a care home for five weeks, but it actually took me six months to fully recover from the operation.

Note 2: Some relatives who put their parent in a care home are able to meet the costs by renting out their parent's empty property.

Note 3: There have been cases where local authorities have wrongly sold elderly people's homes to pay for their **nursing care**. They can only legally do this to pay for their **residential care**. If this has happened to someone you know, advise them that there are lawyers who can help them win compensation on a no win, no fee basis.

Tackling Isolation - Day Centres

Isolation is one of the forgotten problems facing the elderly. It is a problem not really addressed. If an elderly person's only contact is the once a week visit from the nurse, or by a relative bringing their weekly shopping, then they are being deprived of social contact. If an elderly person has to go for four to five days without any contact with anybody, in the long term this can be damaging. We all need social contact with people otherwise we start to lose our social skills. It is easy to forget how to interact with others if our only contact is with professional care people who might only be there for 10 - 20 minutes per week.

This diminution of social skills through isolation can sometimes be mistaken for dementia. Many normal people find it difficult to interact with others, so it is not surprising how someone who is old and has been isolated for long periods, can feel apprehensive and may appear confused when they suddenly find themselves in a social situation where they are expected to interact normally.

Day Centres

Day centres for the elderly are generally funded by the local council. They are places for the elderly to meet and socialise. There are activities for them to participate in and they can even learn new skills. Most have a canteen where hot food is served. When an elderly person is living alone, their everyday social contact can be drastically reduced. Going to a day centre offers them the chance to make new friends and broaden their social circle.

Membership is required to join a day centre, and a nominal fee might have to be paid. The fee will vary from council to council, but to be eligible, the person must be living within the boundary of the local authority that provides the facility.

Many of the workers in day centres are volunteer staff. If trained staff are required for example, staff who are trained to look after those with dementia, there are specialist day centres that are set up to cater for their needs.

If an elderly person is unable to attend a day centre, it is important that their family and friends visit them on a regular basis. These visits will ensure that the person doesn't feel isolated and will help them to retain their social skills.

Day Centres for Respite Care

As mentioned earlier, there are specialist day centres for people suffering from dementia. They allow you to leave the person in the morning and collect them later in the day (usually late afternoon). These centres are popular, so there is usually a waiting list for membership.

Most local authorities will try to provide one day per week respite care; sometimes twice a week if the carer is eligible. If the carer has to be at home 24/7 and does not want to put their charge into a full-time care home, this is a good alternative and gives the carer a break and even a chance to take a part-time job.

Here are some other things which can be done to help combat isolation for elderly people living on their own.

If the elderly person doesn't have family and friends living nearby, there are volunteer groups, often run by a local church, temple or mosque that can organise regular visits.

Frequent phone calls from family and friends are another way of maintaining contact with the elderly person. Not only will they look forward to the calls, they will also enjoy returning the calls without feeling they are becoming a burden.

There are classes run by local colleges where elderly people can learn new skills such as painting, pottery or perhaps, cooking. These are also great places to make new friends and enjoy social interaction.

Watching television can be a good form of stimulus for those living alone. It can become their window to the outside world and reduce any feelings of isolation. It is important to make sure the television is kept in good working order and that it is tuned into their favourite channels. It is also important that the set is placed in a position where the person can watch in comfort. If the person is suffering from dementia, they might forget to tell you that there's something wrong with their television, so regularly check it to make sure everything's ok.

Looking After Yourself

It is important that full-time carers realise that they need to take care of their own health. Time must be made to go for a daily walk or take some other form of regular exercise. Being a carer might only be for a few months or a few years, but often the "job" can be for many years. What is more, the longer the period of caring, the more demanding it can become.

Carers sometimes have to give up their role because their own health has deteriorated. With someone vulnerable depending on their help, it is important for them to look after their health.

Flu jabs should be considered because flu can be very debilitating. Multivitamins should be taken; particularly high doses of vitamin c which can help guard against cold and flu viruses.

A long term carer might lose social contact with people. So it is advisable for them to join some kind of social club or take a hobby where they can meet people. It is easy to forget how to socialise if someone is stuck at home long term. It can even be scary the first time they go out after long periods staying at home; this is especially so when they are meeting people in a formal social setting.

Avoiding Falls - Mobility Aids

Falling is one of the main risks the elderly have to be aware of. Many hospital admissions of older people are due to fractures from falls. Mobility aids are available to help reduce the risk from a fall and to help disabled people get from A to B safely.

The big superstores are now stocking basic mobility aids like wheelchairs and shower chairs. If after assessment, it is established that the person needs some kind of mobility aid, the Social Services can provide it.

If you are planning to buy the aids yourself, they need to be supplied to your specifications to enable you to get maximum benefit. Buying mail order or online is sometimes cheaper, but if you go to a mobility shop, they have trained assistants to make sure the equipment fits your specific needs. Choosing the wrong equipment could cause discomfort or even accidents.

Even a simple thing like an armchair needs to be measured so the seat height is not too low or too high for the user to be able to get up easily. A correctly adjusted chair will help the user maintain good posture. If the user is sitting in their armchair for long periods this is important.

Here is a list of some mobility aids currently available:

Wheelchair - The rims on the sides can be removed if the user is not going to propel the wheelchair themselves; this makes for easier access in tight situations.

Motorised wheelchair - These can be useful on kerbs or steep slopes.

Mobility scooter - A self-drive three or four wheeled buggy.

Zimmer frame - A walking aid where you use both hands to hold the handles.

Commode - A portable toilet; useful if you cannot reach the bathroom easily.

Riser chair - (mechanical) Designed to help you stand up from sitting position.

Riser chair - (motorised) As above but a motorised version. (They can be dangerous with animals and children around). Sadly, a number of children have died after being trapped under these chairs. Pets can also become trapped in the mechanisms. **Note:** My mother's first riser chair started to malfunction and would go up and down by simply tapping the arms of the chair. It is important to be very careful when operating these chairs. Follow the instructions carefully. For safety reasons, the chair should always be switched-off from the mains when not in use.

Shower chair - A chair designed to allow you to have a sit-down shower.

Holding bars - Fixed in corridors or bathrooms to help you keep your balance when walking or turning.

Raised toilet seat – A toilet seat which comes in various sizes from three inches to seven inches. It is firmly attached to the toilet. It raises the toilet seat height to the required level, making it easier to stand up from a sitting position.

Disabled Equipment Specialists

There are few companies specialising in disabled equipment. Below are just two examples. You can go online to find numerous companies who sell disabled equipment.

Web address: www.Betterhealthcare.com
Phone number: 0800 328 9338
Web address: www.otstores.co.uk
Phone number: 0845 260 7061

<u>The Will and Lasting Power of Attorney</u>

The Will

If a person knows who their beneficiaries are they should write a will so that the beneficiaries can receive their estate/capital when the person dies. Otherwise it is usually divided among family members equally unless there is a surviving spouse or partner who will get the whole amount.

Do-it-yourself forms can be downloaded from the Internet or bought from certain high street book shops. These forms are useful if you do not want to go through a solicitor. However, what you write can sometimes be unclear in legal terms and this can lead to others contesting the will. So generally, it is advisable to go through a solicitor.

Lasting Power of Attorney

Granting Lasting Power of Attorney is an important step, especially if you are suffering from dementia's early stages and you can still make decisions. It is basically giving somebody who you trust the right to look after your financial affairs.

Example One: Lasting Power of Attorney is important because if you find yourself suddenly mentally incapacitated and bills have to be paid or other financial transactions need to be made, whoever is looking after you cannot go to your bank and simply say: "I am here in behalf of Mr Smith." Maybe their gas bill has to be paid before they get cut-off. Without Lasting Power of Attorney, the bank will refuse to give you access to the money, however genuine your problem is.

If this happens, the carer should go to The Court of Protection for access rights each time a problem arises. The courts fees are taken from the estate/capital and this can become expensive.

Example Two: If, because of accident of illness, you are put on a life support machine, the decision can be given to whoever has the Power of Attorney to switch it off or keep you on life support.

Note: If you are not happy about giving the Power of Attorney, or cannot fully trust someone, another option is to make a joint account with the person who is looking after you. You can even approach your bank to make a mandate where the person or persons taking care of you have access rights to your money to pay bills. Make sure they can talk on your behalf if there are any problems with your account. Most banks have this facility.

Community Transport Scheme for the Disabled

There is a community transport service for the disabled. It is provided so they can do their shopping or visit friends and relatives. Under the scheme, one carer is allowed to travel with them. Concessions are given for taxi journeys where the disabled person pays a nominal fee for a set mileage. When they exceed the set mileage, they pay the full fee for the journey. There are also community buses for the disabled. Contact your local council for more information on the services they provide, because they tend to vary from council to council.

Freedom Pass

Pensioners are entitled to free off-peak bus and train travel. To receive this benefit, a freedom pass has to be applied for from a local post office.

Disabled Access

Most buses have a disabled access. The bus lowers and a ramp comes out for the wheelchair, but only one wheelchair is allowed on the bus at any one time.

Not all train stations and tube stations are disabled friendly. You need to check before undertaking your journey.

Airports have a wheelchair service if you book it in advance. It can be a long walk from the passport checking area to the plane's departure point. You might even get an express service if you require a wheelchair.

Common Health Problems Facing The Elderly

When we get older our health can sometimes suffer. There are certain illnesses and conditions that particularly affect elderly people; conditions such as high blood pressure, diabetes and arthritis. The following sections are concerned with the most common conditions that can be faced by elderly people.

Doctors do not always fully explain your illness when you go to see them. They just say you are suffering from such and such an illness and here is the medication you have to take. It helps to know a little about what is causing the illness for there to be a chance of remedying it or lessening its effects on your health.

It is good to have a basic understanding of the most common medical conditions affecting the elderly. Hopefully, you will find following the pages helpful. **Please note:** The following information is provided as a general guide only. If you have a genuine concern about a health matter, please seek professional help.

Dementia

Dementia is an illness where the brain is basically ageing to a point where it is not functioning properly. When we are younger, the brain is developing. When we get older the brain is still changing as the rest of the body changes. Unfortunately, this can mean the brain functions can decline as the rest of the body's physical powers decline. Memory loss and confusion are the most common symptoms. When the brain's functionality deteriorates severely, the ability to undertake simple things such as to talk, to walk or eat by yourself, can be lost. People with dementia live on average, 7-14 years after first being diagnosed. 10% live longer than 14 years.

Alzheimer's disease is the most common form of dementia. Early signs are short-term memory loss, confusion and manifestations of stress. Alzheimer's is an incurable, degenerative disease which can be terminal. Medication available can delay the disease if it is suitable for the patient to take, but presently there is no clinically proven cure.

Note: As my mother's dementia started to affect her memory, she would sometimes forget her key when she left the house. Once shut, the door would automatically lock, leaving her locked out. When this happened she had to wait for me to come back from work to let her in. Now her illness has progressed, my mother sometimes becomes aggressive; this was never a part of her character before. Aggression is a common symptom of the disease, and although this can be upsetting for the carer, it should never be taken personally.

Vascular dementia can occur when the arteries carrying blood to the brain are damaged or become thinner because of high blood pressure or diabetes. If the blood cannot carry sufficient oxygen to the brain, the cells can become damaged, which in turn can lead to the onset of dementia.

Dementia is typically a progressive disease - the sufferer's illness gets worse over time. It can have profound effects on the sufferer's character. They might be a very kind and loving person, but because of the illness, they could become violent with mood swings from calm to angry or vice versa; often these mood swings occur without the sufferer being aware of them.

Here Are Five Alternative (non-proven) Remedies:

1) Tests carried out on a small scale have shown that high doses of

vitamin B complex can improve memory. Doctors sometimes provide this to reduce stress - vitamin B is thought to help the nervous system.

2) Turmeric is a spice widely used in Indian cuisine. It is used extensively in the state of Kerala in South India and this is thought to attribute to the low percentage of dementia sufferers in the region.

3) Beetroot juice has properties which help carry oxygen to the blood stream. Tests have shown that drinking 500ml per day can reduce blood pressure. It is thought a good supply of oxygen travelling to the brain can prevent dementia occurring.

4) Mental stimulation is thought to reduce the risks of getting dementia.

5) Exercise increases blood circulation. A good blood supply to the brain can help prevent the onset of the disease.

Diabetes

Diabetes is the inability of the body to produce insulin. This can in turn produce an excess of glucose in the blood stream. This can be dangerous and lead to organ failure. Blindness and strokes are some of the other medical problems facing a diabetes sufferer if they cannot manage control their condition. There are two forms of diabetes. Type One and Type Two.

Best way to manage diabetes is to monitor your glucose level daily.

The readings are taken as millimoles per litre. The ideal reading should be between 4-8mmol/l. You can purchase a diabetes monitor from your local pharmacy to check your glucose levels.

Type One

With type one, the body is hardly producing any insulin, so insulin injections are administered daily to maintain glucose at a normal level in the bloodstream.

Type Two

In the case of type two, the body is not producing enough insulin and either medication is given to maintain glucose at a normal level, or the patient manages to control glucose level in the body by diet and exercise. It might be necessary to take medication if exercise and diet changes are not enough to control the condition.

There was an experiment involving a small number people who managed to self-cure type two diabetes through diet and exercise. However, this was a limited study so the results should be treated with caution.

Four Important Things to Do

1) If someone is diagnosed with the condition, it is important they monitor their glucose levels daily. A glucose reading of between 5-7mmol/l before breakfast is the ideal target to aim for.

2) The feet should be taken care of. They should be washed and moisturised daily and the legs raised from time to time if they become swollen. Infections of the feet can be hard to control due to the diabetes. The gaps between toes should be wiped clean and dried.

Occasionally the toes should be spread to check there are no sores.

3) The eyes should be checked once a year for retinopathy (damage to the retina). Early diagnosis can prevent future blindness. See the article on vision later in the book.

4) A good diet and exercise are essential. If the sufferer is not very mobile, they should be encouraged to perform daily exercises to move their limbs up and down - 10 to 20 times for each limb can make a big difference to their fitness levels.

Osteoporosis

Osteoporosis is a disease that affects the bones. When the bones mineral density becomes very low, the bones are more susceptible to fractures. This is a common problem for the elderly. Usually after 35 the bone density has peaked and starts to weaken. This is a normal a part of getting older.
When we become less active, especially after retirement, osteoporosis can occur. The main problems are when an elderly person with osteoporosis falls - they become more at risk from sustaining fractures. Typically, the fractures tend to be to the wrist and hip. Recovery can be slow, particularly if they have other medical complications.
The best way to treat this disease is prevention. Exercise, even if it is only moderate, is beneficial. (See the section on exercise) A diet high in calcium and vitamin D3 is recommended. (See the section on nutrition for more details). With the right treatment it is possible to reverse this disease.
Avoid soft drinks where possible. The phosphoric acid in most soft drinks can affect the calcium in the bones and make them fragile.

<u>Strokes</u>

When the blood supply to the brain is blocked, damage to the brain cells occurs which can cause:

- Severe headache
- Slurred speech
- Paralysis of one side of the body
- Numbness
- Vision loss or blurred vision

Any of these symptoms could indicate a stroke has occurred. If you notice such symptoms, immediately call 999 or get someone to take you to your local accident and emergency department (A&E) straight away. The hospital will have special equipment which can diagnose if you have suffered a stroke. Fast treatment can save your life and may help you achieve a full recovery.

Note: My mother had a severe headache lasting 72 hours. It was so bad that she could not sleep for two days. All HER GP DID WAS TO PRESCRIBE PAINKILLERS. On the third day she collapsed at home and went into a coma for three days. She had suffered a brain haemorrhage. The neurologist managed to remove brain clot. It took a further three months before she was well enough to come back home. All this could have been avoided if her GP had simply said: "Go to the A& E, you might be suffering a stroke."

Thrush

Thrush is a health condition effecting females. It occurs when unfriendly bacteria build up in the vagina. It can happen to younger people as well as to the elderly. Women with Thrush start to feel pain in the vaginal area accompanied by severe itching. Incontinence can make the problem more likely to occur.

Canesten is a common steroid cream given to combat the condition. It can be purchased from a pharmacy without a doctor's prescription.

Sometimes the pain could be due to high acidity levels in the urine. If this is the case, a medication called Cystopurin taken orally might help. The pharmacist can advise you if the medications available over the counter are suitable for you or if it is necessary for you to consult your doctor first. You can buy a PH testing kit from your local pharmacy to check the acidity of your urine.

Please read the information in the nutrition section covering acidity in food.

Antibiotics are administered for severe cases of thrush.

It is recommended that fluid should be taken on a regular basis so any unfriendly bacteria can be flushed out. If the person is incontinent, their incontinence pad should be changed regularly and the person should be washed. After washing, apply moisturising cream.

Light cranberry juice has properties which are thought to combat urinary infections. The juice can be very beneficial if drunk every day. (Light cranberry juice has less sugar content than the normal cranberry juice)

Podiatry

Podiatry is the diagnosis and treatment of the feet by a trained specialist. The feet can suffer from various problems which if not treated can become painful or dangerous. If you are diabetic it is very important to look after your feet. An infection taking place due to a cut or an ulcer can result in an amputation for a diabetes sufferer. It is important the feet are washed and moisturised daily to help keep them healthy.

Your local health clinic should have a podiatrist attached to it. The basic treatment is to remove hard skin and cut the nails on a regular basis. The podiatrist will treat any fungal infection which might occur in the nails and treat corns. They can also give advice on what footwear is most suitable for you to wear.

If the feet become painful your mobility suffers and you might not be able to exercise. Some problems can be avoided if proper shoes are worn. The long-term wearing of shoes that do not fit correctly can lead to damaged feet in old age.

Orientation

Orientation is important for people who are retired and perhaps do not have any plans for the years of retirement ahead of them. It is a good idea if the elderly person has a calendar at hand so they can keep track of the passing days and months. Reading a daily newspaper is also good for keeping track of events and dates. Newly retired people often miss the daily routines associated with working life, so it is good if they can create new daily routines to replace the old ones.

Perhaps a notice board where the date can be displayed might be useful. They could even be encouraged to use fridge magnet numbers and letters. They could use these for a daily routine of rearranging the magnets to display the current day, date and year. At first it might seem to them to be a bit of a childish thing to do, but it will certainly be beneficial as a routine building exercise.

Filling the house with clocks might also act as a reminder of planned routines at set times throughout the day. Anything that can help give an elderly person a sense of purposefulness and continuity should be considered. It is important that they have enough mental simulation; otherwise they could easily fall into a state of boredom and inertia, where every day simply blends into the next. These suggestions and techniques can work equally well for dementia sufferers.

Oral Hygiene

If the elderly dementia sufferer wears dentures, it is important that these are removed and sterilised every night. In the morning, before replacing the dentures, you should gently brush inside their mouth to remove any build-up of bacteria. Removing bacteria will prevent them from having bad breath. Make sure you thoroughly rinse out the brush after use.

Where the dementia sufferer has their own teeth, regular brushing with a soft bristled toothbrush should be undertaken. Dementia sufferers may not be able to let you know that they are feeling pain, so always be very gentle when brushing their teeth. Regular brushing will help prevent tooth decay, thus, keeping potentially difficult trips to the dentist to a minimum.

Mental Illness

One in four people suffer from mental illness at some stage in their lives. Schizophrenia and depression are common forms of mental illness.

Left untreated, schizophrenia can lead to varying states of psychosis where the schizophrenic can lose track of reality and suffer hallucinations. In severe cases, the sufferer may find the hallucinations extremely frightening.

Depression is a debilitating condition that is characterised by depressed mood, and a loss of pleasure and interest in life. Depression can lead to a sense of hopelessness, which is often made worse by the sufferer's inability to sleep. Clinical depression can last for months or even years and is not the same as feeling a bit down for a day or so. These short term moods swings are all part of the human condition.

For the elderly there might be an increased chance for mental illness due to the following causes:

- Loneliness –A decrease in social circle due to retirement or losing touch with friends

- A loss of purpose or meaning in life - often triggered by retirement

- Bereavement - The loss of partner or spouse

- Health problems - Living with constant pain, reduced mobility due to illness or disability

- The side effects from medications or alcohol

Many depression sufferers fail to recognise that there is anything wrong or remain in a state of denial about their condition. Depression is not a normal part of aging, so it is important that the person seeks professional help. The first step is to contact your GP who may prescribe anti-depressants, or if your condition is acute, may refer you to a specialist.

Over time, many people with mental illness recover naturally or can overcome their condition through self-help. However, seeking professional help in the early stages of mental illness can lead to a much more rapid and full recovery. It is particularly important that schizophrenia sufferers seek immediate professional help. This is a very serious disease and without the correct medication the sufferer can quickly become confused and lose touch with reality.

Kidney Disease

Kidney disease causes the organs to fail to work properly. Kidneys filter the blood to remove unwanted waste products from the bloodstream. High blood pressure and diabetes can affect the kidney's functionality.

If you are diagnosed with kidney problems, provided the condition is not too severe, it is possible through dietary changes to improve the impaired kidneys. A dietician or your GP can advise on special diets which can help improve the functionality of your kidneys.

Here are seven things that are recommended for keeping your kidneys working healthily:

1) Avoid salt. Use herbs and spices as replacement seasonings

2) Avoid food and drink with high potassium levels – for example: bananas, apricots and cola

3) Avoid alcohol

4) Exercise regularly - increased blood circulation will encourage the kidneys to regenerate

5) Drink seven to nine glasses of water daily

6) Be aware of the medications you are taking. Certain medications need to be taken one or two hours apart from other medications. Too many chemicals entering the body at the same time can force the kidneys to work too hard.

7) Ask for a review of your medications by your GP. It is possible that dosages could be reduced or some medications could be deemed to be no longer necessary.

Incontinence

Incontinence is the inability to control the bladder and/or bowels. There are two types of incontinence, urinary and facial. The causes could be because of stress, due to dementia, nerve damage or because the muscles around the bladder have become weakened.
It can be difficult to diagnose exactly why elderly people suffer from incontinence. 30% of women who are over 60 suffer some degree of incontinence. The condition is less common in men.

Common Treatments:

- The first level of therapy is "behavioural management." Alcohol or drinks with high caffeine concentrations (tea and coffee) should be avoided. Caffeine acts as a diuretic stimulating the body to pass water.

- Regular exercise can be undertaken after consultation with you doctor. Exercise especially that which strengthens the lower abdominal and pelvic muscles is very beneficial.

- Absorbent pads are used to combat the consequences of incontinence. Complications arising from incontinence can result in hospital admission. For this reason, absorbent pads are provided through the NHS. **Note:** The NHS only provide a basic supply of pads. If the sufferer's incontinence is severe it might be necessary to buy extra pads from a pharmacy or supermarket.

- A catheter can be inserted into the bladder via the urethra. Urine can then drain freely from the bladder into a bag for collection. This procedure is usually carried out by a community nurse. Long term catheter use can sometimes result in bleeding.

- Medications can be prescribed which will strengthen the bladder.

The acid and bacteria in urine can eat away at the skin. It is important the immediate area is washed and moisturised every time a pad is changed. Rashes caused by contact with urine can become difficult to treat, so it vital to maintain a strict regime of hygiene.

<u>Hypothermia</u>

Hypothermia occurs when the body's temperature falls below 35 degrees. Normal limits are 36.5 -37.5 degrees.
Elderly people are particularly susceptible to hypothermia for the following reasons:

- Their mobility might be limited

- Their appetite may not be good

- They are less aware that they might be cold

- They fail to wear the necessary clothing to keep warm

- They do not set the heating to maintain an adequate room temperature (18 to 22 degrees)

If you think that you may be suffering from hypothermia, call the GP straight away. To keep warm, put on several layers of loose fitting clothes (loose fitting layers of clothing are more efficient at trapping body heat). Put the heating on but don't sit too close to the heat source.

Getting Help

Grants are available to keep your home warm. The roof and walls can be insulated. Draft proof sealant can be put around doors. The government currently give a winter fuel supplement for the over 60s to help them pay their fuel bills. You need to apply to the relevant departments to receive this help.
With rising fuel bills, the cost of keeping warm can be worrying. Pensioners on a tight budget might try to save money by not setting heat levels high enough to protect them from the threat of hypothermia. Wearing extra layers of loose fitting clothing is recommended for keeping the body warm. The head loses most of the body's heat, so wearing a hat in cold spells, especially when going outside, is important. Drinking hot/warm fluids will keep the body warm, but try not to drink too much coffee or tea; replace it instead with herbal tea or warm water from the kettle.

Hearing

Our hearing is very acute when we are younger - we are able to hear a wide range of sounds. However, when we get older our hearing tends to deteriorate. This can cause problems when trying to follow a conversation or when listening to the television or radio.

If you think you might be suffering from hearing loss, go to your GP. He/she will examine your ears to make sure it's not being caused by a build-up of ear wax. If ear wax is found to be the cause of the problem, the doctor (or a nurse) can syringe your ears to remove the wax. A motorised suction method of wax removal has recently been introduced; it is painless, fast and effective. This method is generally carried out by your local clinic or hospital. If your hearing loss is not due to a build-up of wax, your doctor will refer you to a specialist who may recommend that you should be fitted with a hearing aid.

Learning sign language or attending lip reading classes can prove beneficial for people with permanent hearing loss. Technology has been introduced to help people with hearing problems. Most government departments now have a text phone service. To use this service, a text phone has to be purchased and the call charges will be billed separately from your usual telephone service provider.

Here is the contact information for Action on Hearing Loss (As the name suggests, they are a charity run organisation concerned with hearing loss).
Postal address:
19-23 Featherstone Street
London
EC1Y 8SL

Phone:

Information line: 0808 808 0123
Textphone information line: 0808 808 9000
Email address: informationline@hearingloss.org.uk
Website: http://www.actiononhearingloss.org.uk

Visual Problems

If you are over 40 years of age you should have your eyes tested by an optician every two years. Regardless of whether you need spectacles or not, testing can pick up early signs of eye disease and early treatment can prevent the onset of blindness.

The NHS has a national screening programme for retinopathy (damage to the retina). If you are diabetic and over the age of 12, your GP should give you a referral to a health clinic who can facilitate the test. As part of the test, eye drops are placed on the eyes to dilate the pupils. Then photographs are taken of the eyes. The test is pain-free, but the eye drops will make your sight blurred for about 20 minutes. Although the test is not compulsory, a high percentage of diabetics could, as a result of their condition, develop eye disease, so it is important to have this done.

In rare cases the eye drops can cause side-effects such as redness to the eyes, headaches or constant blurred vision. If this happens you need to seek further medical advice.

Blood Pressure

Blood is pumped throughout the body by the heart through arteries. Blood pressure is the measure of the strength the blood is pushing against the blood vessel walls.

Blood pressure is read by two readings or numbers in millimetres of mercury (mmHg) 120/80mmHg means blood pressure is 120 over 80.

The high number is the highest blood pressure when the heart is beating fastest. This is referred to as, systolic. The low number is the lowest pressure when the heart is relaxing. This is called diastolic. It is important to keep you blood pressure low. If it is too high, it can lead to strokes and heart attacks. A high reading would typically be around 140/90mmHg. If your blood pressure is consistently too low it can cause dizziness and cardiovascular diseases. Systolic blood pressure is related to readings under 130mmHg, diastolic blood pressure is related to readings under 75mmHg.

What the Elderly Can Do to Keep Blood Pressure Normal:

- Stop smoking.

- Consume less alcohol. Try alternating days you don't drink to give your body a break.

- Reduce salt levels in food.

- Exercise regularly. Speed walking – at least 30 minutes per day. This form of exercise has become popular for people who do not like the gym and find jogging too strenuous. Exercise in groups or with a partner if possible.

- Try relaxation techniques such as breathing deeply in and out five to ten times per session. Whilst breathing in this way, try to relax all the muscles in your body. Imagine you are floating on air.

- Avoid stressful situations.

Note: Drinking a large glass of beetroot juice daily has been found to reduce blood pressure. The nitrogen in the drink helps carry oxygen to the bloodstream which helps lower blood pressure.

Arthritis

There are several types of arthritis. The common ones are rheumatoid arthritis and osteoarthritis.

Osteoarthritis is basically wear and tear of the joint tissues. The cartilage between the joints wears down and the joints start to rub against each other - causing pain and stiffness. In severe cases the cartilage can be replaced, but your GP will invariably recommend exercise and a healthy diet to strengthen and lubricate the joints. Exercise brings in oxygen and nutrients to the joints which might help regenerate the cartilage. The most common problems occur in the knee joint.

Rheumatoid Arthritis is when the joint tissue becomes inflamed with fluid building up in the joints. It is a chronic disease which can affect all the joints in the body. Scientists do not fully understand why it happens.

Treatments

You should consult your GP so he/she can determine what type of arthritis you have. There are different types of drugs and treatment depending on the type of arthritis. The treatments range from injections and orally taken drugs, to surgery and cutting-edge treatment using stem cell technology.

Self-Treatments

Extra doses of vitamin D, selenium and omega 3 can be taken as a preventative measure. These supplements can also prevent an existing condition from getting worse. Fish oil, olive oil and onions have anti-inflammatory properties. Exercise is always the key. The joints must be kept mobile and muscles surrounding the joints supple and strong. Steady exercise can ease the pain and improve the overall condition. Warming techniques can also relieve pain. Techniques such as taking a warm shower or placing a hot/warm towel on the joints for a few minutes.

Alternative Treatments

Acupuncture has helped some people with arthritis. Massaging mineral oils into the joints to improve the circulation or going to a professional massage therapist may be beneficial.

Thyroid

The thyroid is a gland situated just under the neck. It produces hormones to balance bodily functions. An under active thyroid gland is when the thyroid is not producing enough hormones.

The main symptoms are:

- Tiredness
- Dry skin
- Itching of the skin
- Weight gain

Standard treatment involves taking a hormone producing tablet called Levothyroxine. If not treated, an under active thyroid can cause swelling of the gland, heart disease and mental health problems.

An over active thyroid is when the thyroid gland is producing too many hormones into the bloodstream. It is a more serious condition than an under active thyroid. Some of the symptoms are:

- Hyperactivity
- Weight gain or loss
- An increase in appetite

Treatment is by medication, radiotherapy or surgery. If not treated or managed properly, an over active thyroid can lead to irregular heartbeats which in turn can be fatal.

Pressure Sores

Imagine you are sitting in a chair for two to four hours without getting up. Your buttocks might start to feel sore and your limbs feel stiff with lack of movement. Imagine this is happening all day, every day with you standing up and stretching for just a few minutes every few hours until bedtime.

The chances are you will develop a pressure sore on your bottom or on your limbs where they are in constant contact with the chair. The skin could start to break down because the blood vessels are being closed with the constant pressure. A wound or rash could develop. This is what is called a pressure sore. A person who has very poor mobility and is forced to remain in one position for long periods of time is at high risk from developing this problem. It is recommended helping the immobilised person to stand up (if possible) or move their position every few hours to reduce the risk of pressure sores developing.

If someone is sitting down all day, an attempt should be made to put them in to their bed for couple of hours in the afternoon to elevate pressure on their buttocks. (This is a common pressure sore from sitting down for long periods). This action will also reduce swelling to the legs caused by sitting in the same position for long periods of time.

If the disabled person has to spend long periods in bed, make sure you change their position every few hours from their left side to their right side. To achieve this, put a pillow on the right side of their back then alternate to their left side of their back. Do this every four hours. See the example below.

Alternate the pillow on back to the opposite side every 4 hours.

A pillow can be used to lift the heals off the bed by placing it under the ankles or lower legs.

Special pressure cushions can be purchased to help prevent pressure sores. These can be provided by the community nurse if they think the person is a high risk category.

Extra care should be taken when choosing the type of chair for someone with low mobility. An armchair with cushioned arms is better than one with wooden arms. Wooden arms can cause pressure sores.

Care should also be taken with shoe choice. If the edges of the shoes are in constant contact with the skin, foot protectors can purchased to alleviate pressure points.

Incontinence: Skin which is constantly moist is more at risk of developing pressure sores. Regular inspection of the skin in the areas prone to contact with urine is important.

Pressure Graded Cushions for Chairs

Medium Risk Pressure Cushions

These are cushions filled with "memory" foam. They are pressure graded for low to medium risk patients. They adapt to the contours of the body so weight is distributed evenly.

High Risk Pressure Cushions

These are motorised air cushions. The air is pumped into the cushion then removed in a controlled cycle. It works like a massage machine. The action stimulates blood circulation in the sitting area of the body which reduces pressure sores from occurring in that particular area.

Pressure Mattresses for Beds

Memory Foam Mattresses (medium to low risk)
Just like the cushions, these mattresses adapt to the contours of the body so weight is distributed evenly.

Air Mattresses (high risk)
These are motorised air mattresses where air is circulated into the mattress, then removed in a timed cycle. This action stimulates blood circulation and reduces the pressure on the body areas that are in contact with the mattress.

Air Mattress Overlay

This is an air mattress which works to the same principle as above, but is placed on top of a standard mattress.

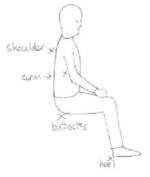

Common pressure sore points on the body.

Pneumonia

Pneumonia is a general term for chest infections and is one of the major causes of death for the elderly. It is sometimes called "the old person's friend" because it's a relatively peacefully way to pass on. This is the illness my mother died from. However, it is not just an illness affecting the elderly; babies and young people are also at risk from pneumonia.

When the chest infection becomes severe, fluid normally starts to build up in the lungs. Respiratory problems occur; fever and coughing are some of the symptoms. When the oxygen supply to the body diminishes to a certain level, confusion, coma and heart failure can occur, eventually resulting in death.

Normal treatment is through antibiotics or vaccines. When the illness reaches a severe stage hospital admission is required. In the final stages, invasive treatment is administered where a tube is put down the lungs to try to pump out the fluid.

Patting of the back or chest very gently from below to the top of the chest and back to loosen the fluid in the lungs is another treatment given in the final stages. It needs to be done for two to three minutes approximately, several times a day, for it to be effective. This treatment can also be carried out in patients with mild chest infections to speed up recovery. However, a doctor should be consulted before undertaking this procedure, and it should be used in conjunction with other treatments and medications. Combined with prescribed medications, this procedure was successful for my mother the few times she caught a mild chest infection.

Sadly, the final time my mother caught a chest infection it didn't help. The oral antibiotic given to her didn't work and the antibiotic given intravenously in hospital also failed to clear the infection. My mother died within five days of catching pneumonia.

Things to do to help prevent pneumonia:

If you are elderly it is recommended that you have an annual flu vaccination.
Wear few layers of clothes to keep warm in winter.
Put on a hat when going out in cold weather and keep the chest area well covered.
Don't eat when lying in bed. It is necessary to sit upright when eating because food particles can get stuck in the lungs which can lead to an infection.

Exercise for the Elderly

Exercise is important for improving the body's circulation and metabolism. This in turn helps keep the body in good health. Exercise is most beneficial if it is combined with eating a balanced diet.

One of the best (and cheapest) forms of exercise is to go out for a daily jog or a brisk walk.

A dementia sufferer will require someone to help them with their exercises. They can have a low attention span so they may need someone to guide them. This is best done by asking them to copy the exercises the helper is doing. It is important to keep the exercise regime fun so they don't lose interest half way through and stop.

Below are set exercises the elderly person can try. Their GP should first be consulted in case they have underlying health problems which might make it unsafe to take exercise. Keep a mobile phone for possible emergencies when exercising away from the home.

Warm-up and Cool Down

All exercises need a warm-up period and a cool down period. The warm-up period might involve keeping the intensity of the exercise low at the beginning then gradually building up until it becomes more vigorous. Cool down is when you decrease the intensity of the exercise. The cool down period should last about three to four minutes before slowly coming to a stop. When you warm up or cool down gradually you are giving your muscles more chance to adapt to the intensity of the workout and also reducing the chance of injury.

Exercise Plan One

Walking briskly for 30 minutes per day is a popular form of exercise. You need to find a suitable route, preferably not too close to a main road. A park might be the best choice because here you will be away from traffic fumes. You should try to go out walking at least four or five time per week to gain maximum benefit.

Exercise Plan Two

Gentle jogging 20-30 minutes per day or every other day will keep you fit.

Just as with the walking exercise, a park could be the best place to jog. If the person you are running with suffers from dementia, crossing busy roads can become dangerous. This is another reason for choosing your local park.

Try to jog with the front part of the feet hitting the ground first. The heel should not be hitting the ground on the first impact – this can cause injury. You will find that it is harder going up an incline so you will need to shorten your stride. On a decline you can increase your stride pattern.

Exercise Plan Three

These are sitting down exercises on a chair, although some of these exercises can also be done standing up.

Firstly, make sure the chair seat height is correct for the person doing the exercise. It should not be too low where the legs are over-stretched or too high where the feet do not reach the ground. For a dementia sufferer, it is necessary to use a chair with arm rests. These could prevent them from falling off the chair if they lose their balance.

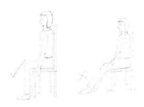

This 15 minute workout should be done daily. Good posture is important. The back should be straight and not slouching.

Clapping for five minutes - You should clap with your hands at waist height. Clap first to your right, then left and then clap with your hands above your head. Try to do this to a rhythm and with a circular movement. After two to three minutes, you can slowly increase the speed of the movements.

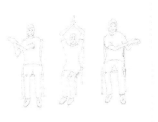

Throwing a ball to and fro with your exercise partner for five minutes. Use a beach ball or a light basketball.

Leg extensions: Kick your left leg out then bring it back. Then do the same with your right leg. Repeat 10 times.

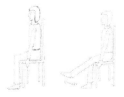

Knee lifts: Lift your knee as high as possible then bring it down. Alternate lifting each knee 10 times.

Roll your shoulder blades five times forward then five times backward.

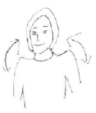

Kick your left foot out then roll your ankle 10 times. Bring it back then do the same for your right leg.

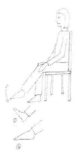

Nutrition and Health

If for whatever reason you are not eating a balanced diet, taking a vitamin supplement will become necessary. If a person with an illness has a deficiency of vitamins, it is likely to hamper their recovery. It is very important for the elderly to ensure that their diet contains all of the essential vitamins to maintain their health. A routine blood test can determine the levels of vitamins and minerals in the body and if there is any deficiency.

Note: I know from personal experience how important to health vitamins can be. Some time ago, I had a problem with a bone in my neck. It started to cause me pain and discomfort. Some days it felt to me that the bone was fractured. After weeks of trying to ignore the problem, I eventually consulted my GP. She suggested that I had a blood test. The test showed that I had very low calcium and vitamin D3 levels. (These are the main building blocks of our bones). Within days of starting a course of calcium and vitamin D3 supplements, the problems with my neck disappeared.

Balanced Diet

It is recommended to eat at least five daily portions of fruit and vegetables to provide essential nutrients. A good way of knowing what to eat is to think about the colours red, yellow and green.

- Red: beetroots, red apples, radishes
- Yellow: bananas, pineapples, lemons
- Green: broad beans, grapes, spinach, celery

Protein

Protein is the body's main building block. Meat, eggs and fish are good sources of protein. For vegetarians, grains, nuts and soya beans are all good sources of protein. A glass of milk can provide 5-7mg of protein and is also high in calcium.

Carbohydrates

Carbohydrates are molecules that the body convert into glucose for energy or to be stored as excess fat. Complex carbohydrates are best for giving the body sustained energy levels, because they take longer for the body to absorb. They are a more stable energy source than simple carbohydrates.

Good sources of complex carbohydrates are brown bread, whole grains, potatoes and rice. Simple carbohydrates are often to be found in processed foods such as biscuits, cakes and doughnuts.

It is recommended the ratio of protein and carbohydrate should be approximately 1/4 protein to 2/3 carbohydrates.

Acidity and Alkalinity Levels

The human body has alkaline and acidity levels that vary in different parts of the body. Our body needs a slightly higher overall alkaline level to maintain good health. Our urine normally has a pH value of 6, while our stomach has a pH value of 1. Overall, our tissues have an acid/alkaline pH level of 7. You can test levels in your urine and saliva by using pH strips which you can buy from your local pharmacy. The normal pH level for urine is 6-6.5. For saliva the normal level should be between 6-7.4.

Note: pH levels are measured from 1-14. A level of 7 is neutral. A level below 7 is considered acidic, and above 7, alkaline.

Try to avoid heavily process foods such as pizzas pasta, bread and cakes. Instead, eat plenty of unrefined wholefoods, such as nuts, grains, fresh fruit and vegetables. Eating too much refined food can raise the acidity levels in our bodies. Lime and lemon can be introduced into your diet to increase alkaline levels.

Acid/alkaline containing foods:

Alkaline	Low alkaline	Acidic	Low acidic
Onions, spinach, olive oil, pears, wild rice, goat cheese, garlic, cucumber, kale	Sesame seeds, cumin seeds, lime, lemons, aubergine, ginseng, tomatoes, watercress	Cheese, cranberries, chicken, tea coffee, soft drinks, beer	Whole grain bread, rye bread, white biscuit, fruit juices

Air Quality

It has been scientifically proven that good air quality is important for our mental and physical health. Elderly people with low mobility, who may have to spend long periods in their homes, should be encouraged to spend as much time as possible in the open air. With the help of a carer, being disabled or elderly should not a reason for not getting access to the great outdoors.

Water

Water is important to our body. We need to drink an adequate amount of water each day so that our body can function properly. At least 7-9 glasses of water should be consumed daily. Elderly people are more prone to urinary infections, so drinking sufficient water to flush out the system, is highly recommended.

Vitamins and Minerals

Vitamins are essential for maintaining good health. Eating a balanced diet will give you all the nutrients needed for a healthy body.

Iron

Iron is a mineral used in the production of red blood cells, or haemoglobin, which is the oxygen-carrying component of blood. Insufficient iron in your diet can lead to anaemia. This condition can be cured by taking an iron supplement. It is recommending that you consult your GP before taking an iron supplement because an overdose can be dangerous.

Iron obtained from eating meat is more easily absorbed than that obtained from vegetables.

The recommended daily intake of iron for people over 50 is 8mg for men, and for 14.8mg for women.

Iron is depleted daily, and not stored in the body like some minerals. Because it is absorbed slowly into the body, it is recommended that orange juice is taken with the iron supplement; the vitamin C in the juice aids absorption. Another way to help the iron absorb more rapidly, is to combine it with a vitamin C supplement.

Good Sources of Iron:

liver	3oz	5.2mg-9.9mg
meat	3oz	2.2mg-2.4mg
Prune juice	3/4 cup	3mg
Lentils	1/2 cup	2.1mg
Spinach boiled	1/2 cup	3.2mg

There are different types of iron supplements. The cheapest is ferrous sulphate which is usually administered by your GP. Side-effects of iron supplements can commonly include constipation or diarrhoea. It might be necessary to experiment with the different types to find which ones suit you best; or reduce the amount temporarily to alleviate the side-effects.

Ferrous Iron Types

Ferrous fumarate
Ferrous sulphate
Ferrous gluconate
Iron supplements come in liquid form or tablets and can be administered through injection by your GP. Injected iron supplements are only administered if the patient suffers from severe iron deficiency. Doses vary from 5mg to 210mg.

Note: The 200mg iron supplement dose usually prescribed by the GP is very strong. The long-term use of high dose iron supplements should be discussed with the GP. If you are taking other medications, the iron supplement should be given at least one hour after or before. This will help absorption and not overwork your kidneys.

Vitamin C

Vitamin C (or ascorbic acid) is an essential vitamin for the body. It plays a vital role in the building and repair of skin tissue, bones, cartilage and teeth. The recommended daily dose for men over 50 is 90mg - for women over 50 the dose is 120mg

Good Sources of Vitamin C:

Orange	1 each	69.69mg
Kiwi fruit	1 each	54mg
Cauliflower	1 CUP	54.93mg
Tomato	1 each ripe	34.38mg
Blueberries	1 cup	18.86mg
Spinach boiled	1 cup	17.64mg
Banana	1 each	10mg

Note: A deficiency in Vitamin C can result in people becoming more susceptible to colds and other infections.

Vitamin B Complex

They are a range of vitamins which are normally found in the same foodstuffs. Vitamin B complex plays an important role in:

- Strengthening the nervous and immune systems
- Cell growth and division
- Promoting red blood cell formation
- Maintaining emotional balance

Some of their benefits are not fully understood yet. Small studies have shown that B vitamins can improve the memory of those suffering from dementia. Some scientists are recommending that people take vitamin B complex supplements from an early age to prevent the onset of dementia later in life. However, this approach has yet to be clinically proven.

List of Vitamin B Complex:

Vitamin B1-thamine
Vitamin B2-riboflavin
Vitamin B3-niacin
Vitamin B5-pantothenic acid
Vitamin B6-pyridoxal
Vitamin B7-biotin
Vitamin B9-folic acid
Vitamin B12-cyanocobalamin

Out of all the vitamins, vitamin B12 is the most complex. It is mainly produced by bacteria hence it is found in meat and dairy foods such as milk, yoghurt and cheese. It can also be produced commercially in laboratories.

Good Sources of Vitamin B12:

Lamb roasted	4 oz	2.45
Liver	1 slice	47
MILK	1 cup	0.9
Fish-trout	3 ounces	4.2

The recommended daily intake for men and women over 50 is 2.4 micrograms.

Note: Vegetarians might be low in vitamin B12, so supplements should be considered.

Calcium and Vitamin D3

These are the main building blocks of bone. When we get older our bone density reduces and we become more susceptible to fractures. A good diet with enough calcium and vitamin D3 is important for keeping bones healthy and strong. (For the same reason, our acidity/alkaline pH levels should be balanced).

Note: Consuming too many soft drinks can be harmful. I was addicted to diet cola. I was drinking several cans every day without realising that the phosphorous in most cola drinks can reduce calcium levels in bones. I found out through a routine blood test that my calcium levels were very low. However, it was only when I was researching for this book that I realised it was because of my addiction to diet cola. Phosphorous is an important mineral for the body but an excess can be harmful. The mineral is found in most foods, so it is rare for someone to be low in phosphorous.

The recommended daily intake of calcium for men and women over 50 is 700mg

Good Sources of Calcium:

milk	1 CUP	300mg
cheese	2 slices of processed cheese	265mg
fish	Salmon canned 75g	208mg
kale	½ cup	49mg

Vitamin D3: Is a vitamin your body can absorb from sunshine, but in our wet and cloudy climate and long winters, our bodies can become depleted. Vitamin D3 works conjunction with calcium to build strong bones.

Vitamin D3 is usually measured in international units (IU).
The recommended daily intake for men and women over 50 is 600-800 (IU) = 15mcg-20mcg

Good Sources of Vitamin D3:

Milk	1 cup	104
Fish(trout)	75g	208
Fortified margarine	2 teaspoon	50
Egg yolk	1	25

Vitamin A

Vitamin A is important for maintaining good vision, especially in low light. It is credited with repairing ageing cells, particularly eye cells. Deficiency in this vitamin can cause dry and sore eyes, dry itchy skin, and leave you prone to infections. In the Third World, a major cause of blindness is lack of vitamin A.
This vitamin comes in two main forms. Retinol which is directly absorbed by the body and beta-carotene which is stored in the intestine and transformed into vitamin A when needed.
If you have to take vitamin A supplements, please note that beta-carotene is safer. A high dosage of vitamin A retinol can be toxic and make you ill.
Good sources of beta-carotene tend to be fruit and vegetables that are orange or yellow in colour. These include: carrots, sweet potatoes, pumpkins, winter squash, apricots, papayas, mangoes and peaches. Animal products such as liver, fish oil and egg-yolk are high in retinol. Liver is very high in retinol and should not be eaten daily, because if retinol builds-up in the body, it could quickly reach toxic levels. Virtually all vegetables and fruit contain beta-carotene; whereas animal products are the main source of retinol.

Vitamin A is usually measured in international units (IU) 1.5mg=5000IU
The recommended daily intake for men over 50 is 3000 (IU) and for women over 50 it is 2330 (IU)

Good Sources of Vitamin A

Banana	1 average size	144IU
Orange	1 average size	405IU
Chicken liver	Cooked 28g(1 ounce)	3732IU
Spinach	180g boiled drained	18867IU

Fatty Acids

Essential fatty acids (EFA) are important for the immune system and for general health.

There are two types of omega fatty acids, omega 3 and omega 6. Omega 3 is considered the more important, but it has to be a balanced with omega 6 for it to be beneficial. Fatty acids need to be ingested because the body does not synthesise its own supply. Nuts and oily fish such as salmon, sardines and mackerel are good sources of omega 3.

Originally, omega 3 and 6 were known as "vitamin F" but research has shown that they are more closely linked to the fats family.

The daily recommended intake of omega 3 should be between 2 grams and 4 grams.

Good Sources of Omega 3

Food	Weight	Omega 3 fatty acid
Walnuts	¼ cup	2.3g
Soybeans cooked	1 cup	1g
Salmon	4 oz	2.1g

Printed in Great Britain
by Amazon